THE LITTLE BOOK OF
ORAL
SEX

First published in Great Britain in 2001

3 5 7 9 10 8 6 4 2

Ebury Press
Random House, 20 Vauxhall Bridge Road, London SW1V 2SA

The Random House Group Limited supports
The Forest Stewardship Council (FSC),
the leading international forest certification organisation.
All our titles that are printed on Greenpeace
approved FSC certified paper carry the FSC logo.
Our paper procurement policy can be found
at www.rbooks.co.uk/environment.

The Random House Group Limited Reg. No. 954009

www.randomhouse.co.uk

A CIP catalogue record for this book is available from the British Library.

Designed by seagulls

Printed and bound in China

ISBN 9780091884772

Papers used by Ebury Press are natural, recyclable products
made from wood grown in sustainable forests.

THE LITTLE BOOK OF
ORAL SEX
for her

EBURY
PRESS

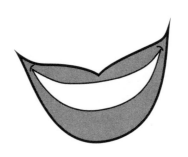

Hello from a champion *cunnilinctor*.

When I was asked to write
this oral manual I was naturally
excited. I'd gone down this road
before in my previous, well-received
hardbacks, *Speaking In Tongues*,
Lick Before You Leap and
Get Your Teeth Into This.

I am more than aware that my
many marriages and countless
sexual encounters the world over
have made me something of a
'cunning linguist'. It is only fair that
I share my profound insight with

as many women as I can –
and as quickly as possible.

Finally, take a tip from me.
What's good for a goose is
also good for a gander. So ladies,
when you've had your fill, why not
let the chaps have a taste?

I like to think this is the last word
on a horny issue. One might
call it my 'gland finale'.

This is your 'orificial' guide. Enjoy!

Frederico Fellatio

Empress Wu Zetian (625 –705 AD) was the only female in Chinese history to rule as emperor.

The Tang dynasty was a time of relative freedom for women.

An autocratic, beautiful and intelligent woman, she designed a custom to symbolically elevate the female and subjugate the male.

All government officials and visiting dignitaries were obliged by royal decree to pay homage to her imperial highness by performing cunnilingus on her.

That's my idea of a Chinese takeaway!

I remember this one wonderful girlfriend with whom I had oral sex – it was so fantastic even the neighbours had a cigarette.

If it's called oral sex
why is it so hard to talk?

I've always thought
of cunnlingus as the
taste of things to come.

Where possible, I would always avoid the following cunnilingus interrupters:

Jalapeño junkies

Hannibal Lecter

Vacuum cleaners

After the Second World War a renowned German fighter ace visited a bordello in New Orleans.

He told the prostitute to do exactly as he ordered: 'First of all, you will take off all your clothes, then you will stand with your legs wide apart and then I will take this cigarette lighter and set fire to your pubic hair.'

The prostitute looked shocked
and asked him, why did
he want to do that?

The Luftwaffe pilot replied,
'When I go down, I always
go down in flames.'

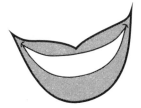

'Never blow in the vagina.'

(Advice from Marty Klein, sex therapist)

I would agree with this although I would suggest you try 'whistling in the vulva' – but only if you know the tune.

An actress friend of mine told
me that she once had oral sex
in a racing driver's Ferrari.

Apparently he went
at a hell of a lick.

They say that shell fish can be an aphrodisiac - well I've always found that 'biting the bearded clam' has done wonders for me!

The three most common lies
made by husbands to their wives:

'Of course I still love you'

'The cheque's in the post'

'I promise not to
come in your mouth'

I've always thought that oral sex
is only 'dirty' if it's done right!

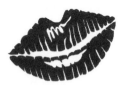

My first wife, Jessica,
was fantastic at oral sex.

Yes, it would be true to say,
'Nothing sucks seeds like ex-Jess'.

'If they didn't show it on the screen, most people would never know about oral sex.'

(Mary Whitehouse, British morality campaigner)

'More taste less speed.'

Some advice for the chaps there

There was once this man
whose tongue was so long that
when he stuck it out for the doctor,
the nurse went, 'Aaaaahhh.'

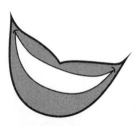

When it's cold, the one thing
that is guaranteed to warm
you up is a spot of 'muff diving'.

I had this girlfriend... well I
got a bit carried away when
performing cunnilingus and she
said she was too embarrassed to
let me do it to her ever again.

I suppose she was
once bitten twice shy ...

A grown-up Little Red Riding Hood was walking through the woods on her way to visit her grandmother when, suddenly, a wolf jumped out from behind a tree. 'Ah-ha!!' the wolf said, 'Now I've got you. And I'm going to eat you!'

'Eat! Eat! Eat!' Little Red Riding Hood replied angrily.

'Damn it!!! Doesn't anybody fuck any more?!?'

A female friend of mine once
said that a perfect lover is a man
with a nine-inch tongue who
can breathe through his ears.

A good tongue is a good weapon.

I'll surrender any time!

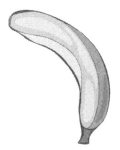

Places I like to come on holiday

Cock Bridge (Aberdeenshire)

Oral (South Dakota)

Head Corn (Kent)

Someone once told me that
you don't have to publicise
oral sex – it becomes popular
by word of mouth.

'The only unnatural sex act is
one which you cannot perform.'

(Alfred Kinsey)

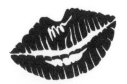

They're changing guard at
Buckingham Palace

Christopher Robin went
down on Alice.
(A.A. Milne)

Better than playing Pooh Sticks!

Now when Snow White
decided to sup

She concocted a good loving cup

Said no to a Coke

Thought Fanta a joke

No – she always
preferred Seven-Up!

GRAFFITTI IN A
LONDON PUBLIC LAVATORY

'I like oral sex with grils.'

Underneath was written...
'Surely you mean girls?'

And underneath that ...
'What's the matter with us grils?'

'How about a quick 68?'

'What's a 68?'

'You give me a blow job
and then I'll owe you one.'

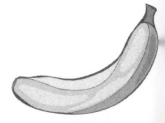

I went out with a farmer's daughter
one summer – she often let me
graze in her meadow.

Plays that failed to excite:

She Stoops to Conquer

The Cherry Orchard

As You Like It

Plays that might have excited:

She Loves To Stoop

The Lady's Not For Biting

That's How I Like It

'The tongue is the
rudder of our ship'

(Adapted from James 3:4)

Talk about a trampsteamer!

'All this fuss about sleeping
together. For physical pleasure I'd
sooner go to my dentist any day.'

(Evelyn Waugh, *Vile Bodies*)

*Now you know why
they say 'Open wide'*

I'm opposed to any sort
of blood sport – although
I have been known to partake
in a little beaver hunting

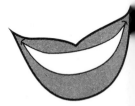

To eat another is sacred.
(John Updike, *Couples*, 1968)

In which case I'm a religious maniac

When I describe a lady
as a 'head turner' I'm not
just talking about her looks.

In Singapore, oral sex is illegal
unless it is a form of foreplay.

**So you're okay for a Fish Head
soup starter if you're following
with meat on a stick – or
Satay as you may know it.**

A couple are in bed.

The husband starts stroking his wife's arm and kisses her on the neck.

The wife turns over and says, 'Darling, I'm sorry but I've got an appointment with the gynaecologist tomorrow and I want to stay fresh.'

The crestfallen husband turns over and tries to sleep.

A few minutes later, he rolls over, nuzzles up to his wife again and whispers in her ear, 'You don't have a dentist's appointment as well tomorrow, do you?'

'If the heart be right, it matters
not which way the head lies'
(Sir Walter Raleigh)

*Alright, so he may have been
at the scaffold but I think
his mind was wandering. . .*

I went out with this oral sex mad
telephonist once – you could say
she was quite a lick operator.

Orchid-eater: 'In the
nineteenth century a gay man,
especially one who enjoyed
performing fellation.'

'The orchid's name is derived from
the Greek word for testicles: *orkhis!*'

Ahhh . . . the scent of a woman.

Ahhh . . . the little petal.

I've always thought that
those who engage in oral
sex have the least to say.

Cunnilingus is the best form
of foreplay – so my advice is,
'Always lick before you leap.'

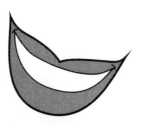

'The kiss originated when the first male reptile licked the first female reptile, implying in a subtle, complimentary way that she was as succulent as the small reptile he had for dinner the night before.'

(F.Scott Fitzgerald, *The Crack Up*, 1945)

The original lounge lizard!

I once dated two women at the same time. Kate was sweet and loving. Edith was feisty and spontaneous. They both loved oral sex and for a while I couldn't believe my luck. But then I had to make a choice between them and I just didn't know what to do. I had to give them both up. I realized that you can't have your Kate and Edith too.

Up until 1980 in Georgia, oral sex –
'a crime against nature' could lead
a practitioner to life imprisonment –
a penalty more severe than having
sex with animals, which in Georgia
was punishable by only five years.

'He that stays in the valley shall
never get over the hill'

*Speaking personally, I'm always
content to 'fall into the ditch'.*

A defeated athlete who later seeks refuge in an oral sex marathon can admit to being well and truly licked.

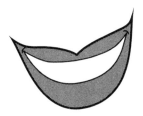

I used to go out with three women
called Cherie. They all loved
cunnilingus. Ahhh . . . in those days,
'Life was just a bowl of Cheries.'

One of my old girlfriends knew
that I loved oral sex and agreed
to have plastic surgery to make it
even better. But then she scrapped
the idea when she discovered that
spare Vulva parts are so expensive.

I've got a hopeless sense
of direction – I'm always
getting lost in my wife's forest.

With delicate fingertips, pinch the arched lips of her house of love very very slowly together, and kiss them as though you kissed her lower lip: this is 'Adhara-sphuritam' (the quivering kiss)

(Excerpt From the Kama Sutra)

Did someone shout 'Bingo?'

'She doesn't have to look
like a model to taste good.'
(Advice from Marty Klein, sex therapist)

I like to have oral sex with
the light on. I always leave
the car door open.

It's a well known fact that
tofu will definitely improve
your sex life – if you can eat
that – you can eat anything.

Familiarity breeds cunnilingus.

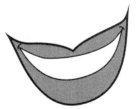

Films that failed to excite me:

The Lady Vanishes

Kiss Me Deadly

A Taste Of Honey

Films that should have worked for me:

La Dulcie Vulva

A Womb With a View

Some Happy Fellatio

In a survey of American women in which they were asked whether they would have sex with Bill Clinton, 98% said, 'Never again!'

Even the Bard is into it . . .

'I have a kind of alacrity in sinking.'

'Done to death by
a slanderous tongue.'

'The play's the thing.'

A Frenchman and an Englishman are hunting in a forest when suddenly a voluptuous, naked blonde races across their path. The Frenchman was immediately smitten: 'Oh she is gorgeous. I would love to eat her.'

So the Englishman shot her.

Soixante-neuf ? I'd say fair
exchange is no robbery.

I don't want to sound big headed,
but, rather cleverly, I can give
oral sex in several languages –
I've actually been described
as a 'cunning linguist'.

'Eat at pleasure, drink at measure.'

And there's nothing more pleasurable than 'shucking the oyster'.

On Grand National Day, a friend of mine was discovered at the Aintree race course under the infamous Beeches Brook jump. He was having oral sex with his girlfriend and was duly arrested. When he appeared in court, the following day, he asked for twenty-five other fences to be taken into consideration.

'Under the tongue men are
crushed to death'

But what a way to go . . .

A GP was asking a depressed
patient about his sex life.

The patient told her, 'When I
get in part way my vision blurs.
And when I get it all the
way in, I can't see a thing.'

'Hmmm.... well, I'm not an
opthalmologist,' said the doctor,
'but would you mind if I
had a look at it?'

So the patient stuck out his tongue.

My second wife was a sex
object but I still had to get
rid of her – every time I asked
for oral sex she objected.

I had this girlfriend who had
all her teeth capped with gold –
I've always found it exciting
to come into money.

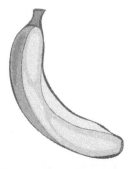

A 1994 sex survey in the US revealed that 76.6% of adult males had performed oral sex, while 78.7% had received it.

Someone's being selfish!

Who said it's better to give than to receive?

I once tried to perform oral
sex on a female financier,
but I just couldn't do it.

I suppose it just shows you ...
there's no taste for accounting.

It's true that Pinky and Perky

Are decidedly kinky and quirky

Down on the farm

They stroll arm in arm

And both like to gobble a turkey

'Last night I discovered a
new form of oral contraceptive.
I asked a girl to go to bed
with me and she said, "No."'

(Woody Allen)

My third wife had a precious metal stud inserted into her clitoris. I liked it – I've always been somewhat partial to 'silver plating'.

'Some men know that a light touch
of the tongue, running from a
woman's toes to her ears, lingering
in the softest way possible in various
places in between, given enough
and sincerely enough, would add
immeasurably to world peace.'

(Marianne Williamson,
A Woman's Worth)

More places I like to come

Maidenhead (Berkshire)

Comers (Grampian)

Cockfosters (London)

I was disturbed the other
night by my wife, Connie,
going down on me.

It was the sort of rude awakening
that I really don't mind.

Bill Clinton is US President.
As Air Force One starts its
descent, the Captain turns on the
loudspeaker: 'We will shortly be
landing in Washington. Mr President,
would you please return the
stewardess to the upright position.'

'Forbid a thing
and that women will do'

(Ovid's *Amores*, 1st century BC)

*Does BC here mean
'Before Cunnilingus?'*

Someone once said that 'the pen is the tongue of the hand'. I think I'll go out and get myself a mammoth magic marker.

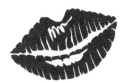

A Koala wants to get laid, so he picks up a prostitute and they check into a hotel.

He goes down on her several times and after they are finished the koala bear starts getting dressed and goes to leave.

'Where's my money?' demands the prostitute.

The koala just shrugs his shoulders and she repeats her request. The koala ignores her.

The prostitute finds a dictionary,
looks up the word 'prostitute'
and points to the part
that says, 'paid for sex'.

The koala picks up the
dictionary, looks up 'Koala'
and shows it to the prostitute.

It says, 'Koala. . . eats bush
and leaves'.

'I think pop music has done
more for oral intercourse
than any thing else that
has ever happened . . .
and vice versa.'

(Frank Zappa)

One tongue is enough
for a woman.
(John Milton)

*But at other times,
it's never enough . . .*

During a particularly passionate
soixante-neuf session with my wife
we both ended up in hospital.
I'm afraid we bit off more
than we could chew.

Did you know that sex has
a speed limit? It's 68 – because
at 69 you have to turn around.

I had this girlfriend who would always laugh when I went down on her and it didn't seem to matter which book she was reading.

A cherry a day
keeps the doctor away

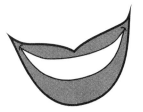

'One half of the world
cannot understand the
pleasures of the other'

(Jane Austen)

As far as I'm concerned
you can forget about going
to restaurants – I'm always
happy to eat Connie's sushi.

In the aftermath of an undercover investigation at a massage parlour by Pennsylvanian State Police, the extent to which officers are supposed to go to 'carry out their duties' is to be clarified following the discovery that two state troopers had actually accepted oral sex.

Police spokesman, Major Ralph Pariandi stated that guidelines need to be laid down, 'Up until now, our people have had to make decisions on the fly.'

Citizens may not enter Wisconsin
with a chicken on their head.

Oral sex is also prohibited.

In other words, 'No Foul Play'.

Oral sex is like a curry –
when it's good . . . it's great
and when it's bad it's still tasty.

I've always thought of
pubic hair as being rather
like parsley - you push it
aside before you eat.

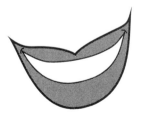

I had a fling with a beautiful musician – a brass player.

Oh how I used to love blowing her vulva trombone.

QUESTION:
What do you call
oral sex between yuppies?

ANSWER:
Sixty something.

Did you hear about the oral sex
mad scientist who was always
desperate to return to the labia?

The Roman poet Martial counsels an ageing friend, 'Why do you plague in vain unhappy vulvas and posteriors; gain but the heights, for there any old member revives.'

'Woe's the wife
that wants the tongue
but well's the man that gets her'

(Scottish Proverb)

There was an old woman
who lived in a shoe

She had so many children
she didn't know what to do

So obviously did she lack
any sense of perception

That it shouldn't perplex
that with oral sex

She could have
avoided conception.

A man with a bad back goes
to his doctor for a check up.

The doctor surprisingly asks,
'When did you last have oral sex?'

The man deliberates a bit and
says, 'Actually I can't remember,
let me just ring my wife.'

He dials home: 'Darling, when did
you last give me a blow job?'

To which his wife replies,
'Who's calling?'

Turnips like a dry bed
but a wet head.

(Vegetarian bumper sticker)

One of my old girl friends
was a really argumentative
during oral sex – she used to
give me a right tongue lashing.

'I'm never through with a woman
until I've had her three ways.'

(John F. Kennedy)

I took one of my girlfriends
out for a ride in the country.

We parked in a secluded
spot and we started to kiss.

All seemed to be going to plan,
but then she said, 'My mother told
me if you pull over into a dark area,
I should say no to everything.'

So, I said to her, 'Would you
mind giving me a blow job?'

I became a devout Christian
once I discovered that
Cunnlingus is next
to Godliness.

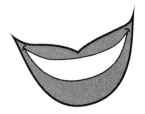

Place your darling on
a couch, set her feet to your
shoulders, clasp her waist,
Suck hard and let your tongue
stir Her overflowing love temple:
this is called `Bahuchushita'
(sucked hard)

(Excerpt from the *Kama Sutra*)

Sofa so good

More cunnilingus interrupters

Chilli Chompers

Jeffrey Dahmer

Bulimics

'If you haven't got a blow job from a superior officer, well, you're just letting the best in life pass you by.'

(Jack Nicholson – *A Few Good Men*, 1992)

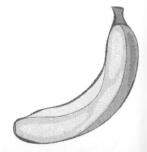

During an interview, when Paula Jones was asked if her experience with Bill Clinton was anything like Monica Lewinsky's.

She supposedly replied 'Close but no cigar.'

'The tongue of idle
persons is never still'

*So laziness really
does beget lewdness...*

I have to admit that
I've got this thing about that TV
horticulturalist Charlie Dimmock.

I wouldn't mind
trimming her lawn.

I've been lucky enough to
'pay lip service' to women from
all over the world and I've
kept a record of some of their
comments afterwards:

GERMAN
I'm glad that's over –
now I can have some food

FRENCH
Now, you'd better leave
quickly before my husband
returns – he's better at it anyhow

AMERICAN
What did you say
your name was?

ITALIAN
At last – something to talk
about in confession.

ENGLISH
I really must do something
about that ceiling.

In Virginia, oral sex between adults – whether homosexual or heterosexual, in public or in private is considered a 'crime against nature' that carries five years in prison.

I'm sure it's very different in the deep south!

More Bed and Bard

'Why, when the
world's mine oyster?'

'O, what men do!'

'Blow, blow, thou winter wind.'

More films that failed to excite:

Scent Of a Woman

The Pumpkin Eater

A Kind Of Loving

More films that would have excited:

Twelve Hungry Men

Quo Vulva

An American In Clitoris

'I've got a PhD in oral sex.'

'Did they make you take any
Spanish with that?'

(Diane Keaton and Woody Allen,
Sleeper, 1973)

If you get bored with
jobs around the house,
let me recommend you
a little `carpet munching'.

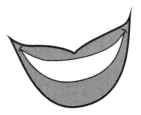

SITOPHILIA

This gastronomic game
is used during bondage.

The male partner is first immobilized,
a paper plate is cut so that a 2"
diameter hole is made off-center.

The plate is held over the male
genitals and these are pulled
through so that they now look
as if they are being served
on a platter.

Spaghetti and meatballs are
served onto the plate and, with fork
in hand, a helpless male is told he
is about to be fed his own balls.

It doesn't matter who eats
the meatballs but each strand
of spaghetti is sensuously
wrapped around the penis
and sucked through the lips
before being eaten.

(Internet 'recipe')

A nice plate of cunnilinguine

Love is a matter of chemistry –
oral sex is a matter of physics.

In Chicago, it is illegal to
eat in a place that's on fire.

*And even if you like
to smoke after sex.*

The Romans had a word for it:

Cinaedus (pervert, one
who submits to oral sex).

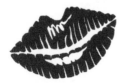

'Descendre à la cave' –
to go down into the basement.

'Brouter le cresson' –
to graze the watercress.

Your first French lessons . . .

An American sexologist
Legman has suggested
that there are 14,288,400
positions for cunnilingus alone.

*Mmm . . . I'm not sure
about this – I've only managed
14,288,399 positions.*

'The proof of the pudding
is in the eating'

Just sago and I'll semolina

A lonely woman is looking
for an unusual pet.

The pet store owner brings
her a frog and says, 'This frog
has been trained to perform
cunnilingus. Just £500.00!'

The woman buys the frog, takes it
home, lies on the floor with her legs
open. The frog does nothing. The
woman angrily returns to the pet
store and complains about the
frog's non-performance.

'Show me what you did,'
says the pet store owner.

So the woman lies on the
floor with her legs open.

The frog just sits there.

The pet store owner moves
over to the woman, puts his
face between her legs, and
yells to the frog, 'All right,
you little bastard, this is the
last time I am showing you!'

The Roman inscription on a mosaic
on the floor before a bench in the
public baths of Ostia reads
statio cunnulingiorum.

This 'cunnilingus stop' was
midway between the men's
and women's sections.

Three men were said to offer the
same service for a fee in Pompeii.

**That must have
got tongues wagging!**

A New York prostitute
picked up a guy who said
to her, 'I want to kiss you
in a place that's dirty.'

So she took him to
Newark, New Jersey.

In a 2001 internet survey
16% of females interrogated
had never had their watercress
grazed but 49% had enjoyed
it with another woman.

'There is more than one
way to skin a cat.'

Or even boil the bunny

Chaucer – The Miller's Tale:
'Abak he stirte, and thoughte it was
amys, /For wel he wiste a womman
hath no berd. /He felt a thyng al
rough and long yherd, /And seyde,
'Fy! allas! what have I do?'

*That's quite a mouthful!
But this is the earliest literary
reference to the discovery by
chance of oral sex – In other
words, 'the accidental birth
of a cunnilinguist'*

What do performing
cunnilingus and working
for the Mafia have in common?

Just one slip of the tongue...

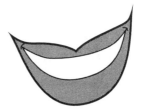

'French Culture' is
prostitutes' slang for oral sex.

Bill Clinton asked Monica if she'd like to see the Presidential clock.

She of course replied yes.

He unzipped his trousers and let it all hang out.

Shocked, Monica screamed, 'But that's not a clock!'

Bill replied, 'It will be when you put two hands and a face on it.'

How did the slave
feel after pleasuring
the Roman Emperor's wife?

He was gladiator.

'Gobble one's goofy' is
an Australian euphemism
for cunnilingus.

That would make you
go down with a smile!

I knew this WREN whose nickname was Titanic - it seemed she was always going down with the captain and crew.

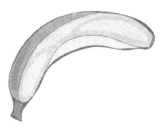

Aural sex should be heard
but not obscene.

Did you hear that Continental
Airlines are planning to merge
with Air Lingus to form
Conilingus Airlines?

Further mouthwatering places

Lick (California)

Tongue Point Village (Oregon)

Sucker Flat (California)

'Dip me in honey
and throw me to the Lesbians'

(US bumper sticker)

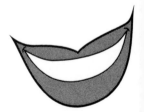

In Montana it is illegal for
a man and a woman to
have sex in any other
position than missionary fashion.

**So, no bad mouthing
in Montana, then.**

I used to be teacher but I'll never go back to it – I'm much happier now that I've moved from the public sector to the pubic sector.

If oral sex didn't exist,
all the money in the world
would have no meaning.

'GOING DOWN . . .
GOING DOWN . . .
GOING DOWN'

(Crowd chant heard at
football grounds all over the country)

I'm not that wild about fruit –
although I do like chewing cherries.

Let your tongue rest for
a moment in the archway
to the flower-boughed Lord's
temple before entering to
worship vigorously, causing her
seed to flow: this is 'Jihva-mardita.'
(the tongue massage)

(Excerpt from the *Kama Sutra*)

Amen to that!